Losing Belly Fat and Weight Quickly: The Best Recipes For Shredding Fat

All rights Reserved. No part of this publication or the information in it may be quoted from or reproduced in any form by means such as printing, scanning, photocopying or otherwise without prior written permission of the copyright holder.

Disclaimer and Terms of Use: Effort has been made to ensure that the information in this book is accurate and complete, however, the author and the publisher do not warrant the accuracy of the information, text and graphics contained within the book due to the rapidly changing nature of science, research, known and unknown facts and internet. The Author and the publisher do not hold any responsibility for errors, omissions or contrary interpretation of the subject matter herein. This book is presented solely for motivational and informational purposes only.

Table of Contents

Toast Topped With Almond Butter 30

Lentil Soup With Pita Bread 31

Almond And Banana Shake 32

Egg And Brown Rice Salad 33

Introduction

Losing weight is one big task for an obese person. The body fat basically consists of three layers of fat.

Body fat

Muscle fat

Body Water

When someone starts with the diet process and starts working out then the first thing that one loses, without much effort, is body water. It is formed in the body when exercise is missing in someone's routine. After some efforts body loses muscle fat, the excess of carbohydrate that is present in muscle. The most difficult layer to lose is the actual fat content in the body. This is the stable fat of the body and is very difficult to lose. It takes persistent efforts to lose some fat content of the body. Once someone looses this fat from the body and the person leaves the workout for some time then also this fat layer does not built up. Whatever fat is built up that is muscle fat only. Apart from workout it is very important to take care of one's diet. Proper diet supplements the process of workout. If one takes oily and fatty diet then the body workout will not help to lose the body fat. The intake of fatty acids will have to be reduced from the diet and then only the excess reserve of fat will be lost. One has to plan the diet accordingly so that the body is not drained out of energy and the body also loses fat content.

The body will have to take proper protein content in the diet so that the body supplies the essential muscle making content to the body.

The diet will have to be balanced in terms of less carbohydrates, no fats, and lot of protein content, minerals and fibers.

One needs to take some food just 30 minutes after the workout to supply essential protein content to the body and help in making of muscle.

Fiber content is very important in the body. Fiber is one important factor which maintains the body water in the body. One, who is working out, sheds a lot of water and salt during workout. It is important that body retains water otherwise body will dehydrate during the workout process. So the balance diet will have to include the fiber content in the diet. Fiber contains the roughage which though does not provide any nutrient but helps in retaining of water into body.

One can make healthy recipes and make the diet balanced and proper. The recipes mentioned below can be prepared with in less than 30 minutes and are good in eating.

Table Cheese Omelet With Broccoli

There are two components in this dish one is the egg omelet and second is broccoli. Broccoli gives fibers content to the body and egg omelet is rich in protein content. This protein rich content fill the stomach with protein and does not leave any space for the carbohydrates intake. This is one healthy way of eating as it balances the diet and also provides supplement for growing strong muscles, which tears down after heavy workout. This dish can be eaten in breakfast and is sufficient to keep stomach full for 2-3 hours. The calorie in broccoli is also less, just 30 calories.

Salad Noodles With Salmon

The main components of this dish are the salad contents; asparagus, avocado, boiled veggies, salmon and noodles. The salad, boiled veggies and asparagus will give proper mineral content to the body. They contain vitamins like A, and vitamin B. Minerals are also present like iron. The salmon content and the avocado will provide healthy fats to the diet which will provide energy to the body. This energy will help in doing proper workout. The last but not the least, noodle in veggies will provide the required fiber to the body. This fiber will hold the body water and salt in the body.

Banana Pieces Dipped In Chocolate

There are some healthy carbohydrates which are good for body and they help in easy break down of calories and also insist body to eat less. These kind of healthy carbohydrates are very important for body to have proper energy content in body. Banana is a rich source of resistant starch which is a basic nutrient of healthy carbohydrates. Chocolates are known to be the rich source of MUF's. MUF's helps in the activation of metabolism process in the because of which the fat losing process starts. MFU is a content block of healthy fats, which again are good for body. This recipe becomes a complete diet with the presence of healthy carbohydrates and healthy fats. It can be taken in lunch time so that body does not become energy less.

Baguette Sandwich With Blackberry Salad

Baguette is a French thin and long loaf of bread. It basically contains lot of carbohydrates and some proteins and some essential amount of fats. It forms the base of this recipe which provides energy to the body. Blackberry is a fruit which contains minerals and vitamins. Blackberry contains antioxidants which help in stopping of oxidation process of certain elements in the body. Antioxidants when taken in high amount it helps in prevention of cancer and also slows down the ageing process of the body. Apart from antioxidant, it also contains vitamin C and vitamin K and many minerals. It contains fibers which helps in the digestion process and maintains a proper bowel moment of the body.

Chickpea With Fat Free Yogurt And Slaw

Slaw is the shredded cabbage. This contains a lot of soluble fiber in it and it helps in water retention of the body. Chickpea is a kind of pulse which has to be properly washed and rinsed. This contains a lot of protein content again helpful for the muscle growth in the body. It also contains resistance starch which provides energy to the body without getting deposited in the muscles to form fat. Fat free yogurt contains the essential and important fats. This recipe can be taken in lunch and one will have a filled stomach till dinner.

Banana And Grapefruit

Grapefruit in itself a good option for breakfast when someone is on a diet plan. It can also be taken as a side fruit in brunch. This is one fruit which contains maximum amount of water in it; almost 90% of the fruit is water. When one has this fruit, the stomach gets filled in very less time and the person does not feel like having anything else for breakfast. The juice of the fruit fills up the stomach completely and thus over eating is avoided. It is considered as the best weight loss food. This is basically because it affects the insulin content of the body. Insulin, in body, helps in storage of fat into the body. Banana adds the fiber content and mineral content to the overall diet. It adds dietary carbohydrates to the overall dish.

Chili Red Kidney Beans

This is one dish which contains two ingredients which affects the fat directly and helps in burning of the same. The dish has red kidney beans and chili powder. The red chili powder contains capsaicin, this is the main nutrient found in chili and it heats up the body when taken. This heating up burns a lot of calorie in the body and also burns the stored fat content of the body. Kidney beans, on the other hand, are protein rich food. It contains full for of proteins. The combination of the two makes this dish a fat burning dish. The dish also contains a lot of herbs and spices. This adds on to the burning feel that this dish gives. It takes about 45 minutes to prepare the dish and can be eaten in dinner or lunch.

Healthy Turkey Burger

The people who are used to eating a lot of beef, which contains a lot of fat, now have an alternate to the beef burger; turkey burger. Turkey is grilled with garlic and cumin, in form of patties, and is put inside the bun to become the dish. Turkey has lot of lean protein and it helps greatly in fat reduction. They contain amino acid which is the basic blocks which builds muscles. When a person takes turkey, it is quite fulfilling and sustains till dinner, when taken as a lunch.

Rice And Salad

Brown rice when cooked with chickpea and dates, in olive oil, it becomes a fulfilling dish which can be had in lunch as well as dinner. Dates are a great source of fiber and hemoglobin. People who are anemic in nature, have a problem in reducing fat and are also not able to work out for longer duration because of less oxygen supply to the cells. Taking dates help anemic people greatly. Brown rice, again, contains very less amount of fatty starch and basically has good starch content which gives energy to the body. Chickpea also contains resistance starch and pure form of protein which helps in building the muscles. When the prepared rice is taken along with some salad, then it is really tasty and fulfilling for stomach and is also rich in minerals, fibers, protein and healthy starch.

Meatless Quinoa

Quinoa is a whole grain which is grown in South America and is a rich source of protein and fiber. This is one perfect combination to maintain one's energy and start the process of metabolism and build the muscles after workout. One can take this dish after workout, probably in lunch. It can also be taken as side dish with main course, in dinner. Quinoa is cooked with black beans, green veggies and some herbs to give a perfect aroma to the food. Black beans are a great source of fibers and veggies are a source of minerals and vitamins. It is a perfect combination of all the nutrients that a body needs. Meat Quinoa becomes very fatty but when it is without meat, it still gives a perfect blend of taste. The dish contains a lot of energy.

Banana Mixed In Sunflower Seeds

To get a satisfying meal in breakfast, apart from oats, switch to boiled barley and bananas. Banana when taken with barley forms nearly 8 grams of resistance starch and also produces fibers which are rich in starting metabolism process. One can pour in some honey and some sunflower seeds to make the dish tastier. It takes hardly 10 minutes to prepare the dish and also the time taken to cook barley is the only cooking time. The barley is not supposed to be overcooked just a quick cooking will do. One should avoid taking any salt, in the dish.

Healthy Parfait

Parfait means the frozen food which has many layers of fruits, cream, yogurt and some sugar. Healthy parfait does contain layers of food but the layers are all healthy in nature. It contains layer of dates, fruits, yogurt, cereals, plums and peaches. To garnish the dish a bit one can add some walnuts and almonds from the top along with some honey. The dish is a perfect one for breakfast. When the whole scoop of all the layers is eaten together it gives a wonderful taste and is also rich in various healthy nutrients like resistant starch, minerals and fibers. The preparation time of the dish is also very less.

Chilled Green Tea

Green tea has a lot of fat burning properties. It contains an element known as EGCG. It starts the metabolism process and burns the fat rapidly into the body. It is said that if one takes green tea, four times a day, regularly then one can reduce upto 8 pounds in a few weeks. To make chilled green tea one needs a glass full of chilled green tea, some fat free yogurt, any fruit like peach or pear, some drops of lemon juice, and some ice cubes. When all the ingredients are mixed and blended then it gives a rich and healthy smoothie. The person who is now bored of sipping in hot green tea, can for once, switch to the above mentioned smoothie. It is a perfect morning breakfast one can ask for.

Spinach Sandwich In Egg Salad

To eat something tasty, healthy and protein rich one can always turn to eggs. A person can have egg in numerous ways and in all the forms egg taste really well and the richness is maintained. Make an egg salad by cooking it hard and then cutting it in cubes. Mix some red bell pepper, some curry powder and some yogurt. Put this paste on the rye bread topped with spinach leaf. This whole dish is rich in protein content, rich in resistant starch as that is the main component of rye bread used here. Spinach is a great source of iron and curry power adds on to the metabolism process by shooting up the heat level of the body. A dieter cannot ask for more than this; a perfect combination of health and taste.

Chilaquiles

Chilaquiles are a perfect Mexican food which is made out of corn tortillas. Chilaquiles when cooked in a healthy way proves to be a real fat cutter food. To cook this dish one needs oven as there are various layers of food that has to be cooked together. First layer consist of corn tortillas and second layer consist of shredded and boiled chicken breast. This chicken is a rich in protein content and has lot of muscle building blocks. The recipe, if was fried then it would have turned into a fatty food. Rather than frying the dish, we have baked it in oven and because of baking the taste of the dish remains intact and also becomes less fatty for the dieters.

Black Bean Soup

The process to cook this soup is very simple. One has to cook black beans in onions and has to use chili powder and jalapeno. Now the main point here is that, chili powder and jalapeno are so spicy and reacts rapidly into the stomach. They start the metabolism process rapidly. Along with the chili effect, we are making a combination of black beans. Black beans are the richest source of pure protein content and also contains a lot of fiber. Now this tasty soup serves as a real fat cutter and muscle builder. One can use some garlic flakes, some cumin powder and some cream to give an added taste and aroma to the dish.

Avocado Chips

It just is so simple to pick one chips and pop it down the mouth even without giving a thought that how much calorie intake is being done in just one chip. One just has a habit of eating it in the snacks time after lunch. We have a perfect replacement of the fatty chip. We can make avocado chips which can form a great source of evening snacks. Avocado contains oleic acid. This oleic acid helps in the production of oleoylethanolamide in the small intestine. This is the main source through which the brain gets a signal that the stomach is full. So in short, avocado helps in reducing the craving for food and thus helps in avoiding over eating. Especially it helps in avoiding junk food like chips.

Grilled Salmon

Salmon is a kind of premium fish rich in protein content and has monounsaturated fat. Monounsaturated fat, after research, has been proven to have properties which help in reduction of unwanted fats in the body. Salmon also contains lean protein which again is the building block of any muscle in the body. Apart from the mentioned two nutrients, it also contains fats which are healthy for heart. This fat is known as omega 3s. It is pretty simple to cook the salmon, just insert a fork to see if the fork passes the meat easily. Top salmon with some pineapple salsa and have the food.

Italian Chickpea Salad

This is a pure vegetarian dish with many benefits for health. It belongs to Mediterranean diet and has proven to be a real healthy diet. It contains feta cheese which is also known with other name as Greek cheese. It contains lot of protein and has low fat content in it. The salad contains some veggies like tomato and onion to make the diet vitamin rich and had chickpea which is a great source of lean protein. With one full cup of this salad one gets only 160 calories and a lot of other fat reducing and muscle building nutrients. This is not at all a bad call to start the day with.

Grapefruit And Raw Kale Salad

Grapefruit is one great source of fat cutter. It contains fruit juice which gives a signal to brain that the stomach is full. The main content of grapefruit is water so it is fulfilling and a proper dietary food in itself. When grapefruit is mixed with raw kale, a green leaf, it makes it a perfect combination of fibrous food. Green leaf contains lot of vitamin A, vitamin C and vitamin K in it. One can even put some hazelnut pieces in it to give a good aroma and taste to the salad. The food helps in bring the bad cholesterol level down, in the body.

Oat Dipped In Chocolate

One need not remain away from deserts to reduce the fat present in the body. They can have chocolate along with honey and some other healthy cereals to make a perfectly delicious and healthy desert. The three main ingredients of this dish are chocolate, oats and peanut butter that hold the chocolate with oats. Peanut butter apart from acting as a glue also contains some important protein which helps in muscle building. Dark chocolate is a rich source of unsaturated fats which helps in curbing the need for food and oats are a perfect source of fiber and resistance starch, which provides energy to the body. One just has to take the three items in a bowl and mix it with the help of some low fat milk. It becomes like a thick paste which can be made into the shape of a ball and thus have it.

Avocado Spread

To give the fat conscious people a perfect spread for their sandwich, we have a recipe for them. Avocado is supposed to have lot of monounsaturated fat which speeds up the metabolism process in the body and also keeps the stomach full for some time. Monounsaturated fats are nothing but essential fatty acids which are good for body and decrease the bad fatty acids from the body. It is very easy to make avocado spread. Take avocado and peel it and cut it. Mix it with some Tahini and some pepper and salt. Grind it in the processor and sprinkle some pepper onto it. Put some lemon juice in it and cover it with a cloth. Use the spread in sandwich and get a tasty fat free diet.

Toast Topped With Almond Butter

Almond butter is a rich source of healthy monounsaturated acid and also had proteins which is fulfilling in nature. When that is topped with the rye toast then it becomes a perfect combination of proteins, resistant starch and fiber. Top the mixture with yet another fruit; banana. Banana will add on to the resistant starch content of the dish. It will help boosting the metabolism process of the body. One should have just two slices of this dish and then, because of hunger curbing protein content the person feels full till lunch time.

Lentil Soup With Pita Bread

Pita bread is a kind of bread made out of wheat. This is round shapes bread and has lot of resistant starch in it. Lentil soup contains lot of lentil in it which is a very rich source of protein content. It is said that if a person had one bowl of lentil soup his daily need of protein is fulfilled to one third amount. It takes just ten minutes to make the dish. One can add some carrot, some celery and some lemon juice to the lentil and boil it in 8 bowls of water. Bake the pita bread and serve it as bread with the soup. This is fulfilling and one will not need to take anything for next 4-5 hours.

Almond And Banana Shake

Almond is rich in monounsaturated fat and banana is rich in resistant starch. This can prove as best drink just after workout to give proper supply of proteins to the muscle and help in the muscle building. One just needs to grind banana slices with almond milk and pour in some honey and cardamom from top for some good aroma. Put in some ice cubes and drink the tasty and healthy throat chilling drink.

Egg And Brown Rice Salad

The dieters should never forget the intake of egg in their diet. It is tasty and protein rich food. Mix the par boiled egg pieces with the cooked brown rice and get a perfect combination of resistance starch and lean protein in the diet. This can be taken in lunch after workout to give a proper supply of protein to the torn out muscles.

www.ingramcontent.com/pod-product-compliance
Lightning Source LLC
Chambersburg PA
CBHW061944280526
45787CB00004B/1716